The Keto Diet Made Simple

THE CLEAR

2 WEEKS KETO DIET PLAN

TO BURN FATS AND FEEL AMAZING

STEVEN G. CANTY

© Copyright 2017- All rights reserved.

The follow eBook is reproduced below with the goal of providing information that is as accurate and reliable as possible. Regardless, purchasing this eBook can be seen as consent to the fact that both the publisher and the author of this book are in no way experts on the topics discussed within and that any recommendations or suggestions that are made herein are for entertainment purposes only. Professionals should be consulted as needed prior to undertaking any of the action endorsed herein.

This declaration is deemed fair and valid by both the American Bar Association and the Committee of Publishers Association and is legally binding throughout the United States.

Furthermore, the transmission, duplication or reproduction of any of the following work including specific information will be considered an illegal act irrespective of if it is done electronically or in print. This extends to creating a secondary or tertiary copy of the work or a recorded copy and is only allowed with express written consent from the Publisher. All additional right reserved.

The information in the following pages is broadly considered to be a truthful and accurate account of facts and as such any inattention, use or misuse of the information in question by the reader will render any resulting actions solely under their purview. There are no scenarios in which the publisher or the original author of this work can be in any fashion deemed liable for any hardship or damages that may befall them after undertaking information described herein.

Additionally, the information in the following pages is intended only for informational purposes and should thus be thought of as universal. As befitting its nature, it is presented without assurance regarding its prolonged validity or interim quality. Trademarks that are mentioned are done without written consent and can in no way be considered an endorsement from the trademark holder.

"Let food be thy medicine and medicine be

thy food"

Hippocrates

Table of Contents

Introduction 1

Chapter One
   Ketogenic 101 2

Chapter Two
   Getting Started 11

Chapter Three
   Meal Plan 19

Chapter Four
   Keto Kitchen Hacks 45

Chapter Five
   Tips for Maximizing and Maintaining a Keto Lifestyle 55

Conclusion 65

Introduction

Congratulations on taking the first step toward a healthier life! You are going to learn an incredible wealth of information in an easy and understandable way. This book will break down everything you need to know about a ketogenic lifestyle including meal plans, what to avoid and kitchen hacks to make going keto as easy and comfortable as possible.

Whether you are brand new to the ketogenic theory or have tried it before unsuccessfully, this book will be your go-to for all the things you need to know about keto and your companion as you go through your journey.

We will begin with ketogenic 101 and explain every facet of the diet and answer all the questions you might have as you begin.

We will then provide food lists including what to avoid and a comprehensive two-week meal plan full of simple meals that anyone can make. At the end of the book, you will find useful tips for grocery shopping, in the kitchen and even what to do if you are eating out!

I truly believe that the ketogenic diet is the best thing you can do for your health and am thrilled that you have chosen to start your journey with this book.

Chapter One
Ketogenic 101

What *is* ketogenic?

"Nutritional ketosis is an amazing tool for reversing disease processes including inflammation, diabetes type 2, autoimmunity and even cancer growth. It is a serious medical tool which can be used to improve health while allowing the patient to be their own manager."

Dr. Toni Bark, M.D.

Not to be confused with ketoacidosis, which is a bad liver issue that typically affects diabetics and alcoholics, ketogenic means that your body is in a metabolic state that produces a high amount of ketones (main source of energy for the body and brain) and is burning fat instead of carbohydrates. The state of ketosis is achieved when the body is out of carbohydrates so it burns fat instead. We can accomplish this by starving our body of carbs and increasing the amount of ketones we produce. In other words, the ketogenic diet is a low-carb, normal protein, high (good) fat nutritional lifestyle.

The Science of Keto

Not everyone is a science whiz so let's keep this section as simple and easy as possible. Knowing the how and why of keto is important so you can understand what exactly you are doing to yourself and why your body is working the way it is.

Our bodies need fuel and in this day and age, we are bombarded with boxed meals and quick fixes for energy. Processed sugar, bread, cereal, meal bars and carby snacks are easy and cheap. When we hit that afternoon slump it is easy to grab a candy bar or bottle of soda for a quick boost of energy. The problem is that sugar and carbs stay in our bodies and turn into fat, elevate our blood sugar and turn us into overweight, pre-diabetic people. Our bodies have become inefficient at burning fat because they are overloaded with carbs that they can't really use. Carbs are only efficient for athletes who require more fast-acting energy and they are burnt off immediately. So unless you are planning on running a few miles after you eat that bowl of rice or pasta, all those carbs and sugars are going to stay in your body and turn into insulin which stores fat for energy.

But, don't our brains need glucose for good function?

Yes, our brains do require a very small amount of glucose to function properly. However, when we get enough protein and fat it can produce the right amount of glucose for our brain. Also, ketones are actually the main source of energy for our brain and body so making sure we are producing enough ketones is vital. Most people are ketone-deficient which is why we feel sluggish in the afternoon and fatigue has become a common chronic condition. Sugar and processed carbs are directly responsible for the crash and burn lifestyle.

What are ketones?

Ketones are energy molecules that are produced for energy when our bodies are running on low carbs and then low insulin levels, they take the place of glucose in a majority of the instances where glucose is broken down for energy. In the few cases where no glucose supplements will be accepted in the body, fat is naturally changed into glucose and used for those purposes.

Our bodies and brains can very efficiently run on fat so when we have a surplus of ketones available, our brains and bodies use (burn) them for energy. When there are enough ketones present it is a good indicator that we are low on insulin and thus in a high fat-burning state. Ketones are easy to measure with test strips widely available for purchase at almost any drug store and online.

Types of Keto Diets

There are four types of ketogenic diets. **Standard, cyclical, high protein** and **targeted.** The standard and high protein styles are the most common. The standard keto diet consists of a normal amount of protein and a ratio of **70% fat, 25% protein** and **5% carbs**. The high protein method is more like **60% fat, 35% protein** and **5% carbs**. The cyclical and targeted methods are generally used by bodybuilders and athletes and are more advanced. The cyclical keto diet includes 1-2 days of carbs (called "re-feed days") and the targeted method includes added carbs around workouts. The standard and high protein diets are also the most studied keto diets.

Why Should I Go Keto?

There are so many diets out there that it's difficult to choose the right one. The problem is that most diets are just a temporary solution to a complex issue that can't be fixed with a few weeks of restrictions, deprivation and calorie-counting. People are almost guaranteed to fail because with deprivation comes cravings and desire which we all give into eventually. Then we think we have failed so we just give up completely. Diets are not sustainable. They don't teach you how to change eating habits for the long-term. **Keto is a lifestyle**.

Weight Loss

Since 2002, over twenty human studies have been done on low-carb diets. People have always believed that a low-fat diet was the best way to lose weight. However, research shows that those on a high-fat, low-carb diet lost over two times more weight. As mentioned before, our brain and body needs fat for energy so if we are depriving ourselves of that good fat, what happens? Our energy drains and we become dependent on carbs, sugars and chemicals for energy.

With the increase in carbs comes an increase in triglycerides (stored fat), belly fat, insulin levels, blood sugar and other chronic problems. Not only that, but low-fat products are usually highly processed and include a lot of chemicals and fillers to make them look and taste good. Skim milk is dyed white because it is gray once all the fat is taken out. Not only that but when fat is taken out of dairy, the most valuable part is removed.

Many diets leave us with excess visceral (belly) fat. This is because they are not high enough in good fat. Visceral fat is not only the most stubborn but it is also the most dangerous. I like to call it "diabetes belly" because it is directly linked to high-carb, high insulin diets. Keto has been shown to be the most effective diet for belly fat loss. It may seem odd to hear someone say "Eat more fat for your fat belly!" but it works.

As your triglycerides go down, your levels of HDL (High Density Lipoprotein) which moves cholesterol from your body to your liver where it can be broken down or excreted.

Inflammation

Another invaluable side effect of going keto is the elimination of inflammation. Inflammation is your body's response to stress. While this does include mental, emotional and environmental stress, it can also be caused by food and diet.

Food allergies and sensitivities, imbalance of bacteria and fungi in the gut, and too much sugar, carbs, trans fat and protein (especially animal protein) directly causes inflammation. Inflammation is the root cause of an ever-growing list of chronic diseases, syndromes and autoimmune disorders. Some of these include: cancer, allergies, heart disease, diabetes, chronic pain and fatigue, candida, arthritis, psoriasis, acid reflux, digestive issues, high blood pressure, susceptibility to infections, urinary tract infections and more. Eliminating inflammation will usually also eliminate many other issues as well.

Type 2 Diabetes

People with type 2 diabetes have what is called "insulin resistance." In other words, when healthy people eat, their bodies produce a hormone called insulin which tells the body to either store or burn glucose. However, for those with diabetes, their cells don't "recognize" the insulin so the glucose stays in the blood stream

When a type 2 diabetic cuts carbohydrates, the blood sugar and the need for insulin decrease to a save and healthy level. In one study, 95% of type 2 diabetics were able to get off their insulin within 6 months of cutting carbs.

You should always consult with your doctor before trying any diet or making any changes to your treatment.

Paleo, Atkins, Keto, Low-Fat, Mediterranean...?

It seems that every year there is a new fad-diet. Doctors on TV are constantly promoting the latest diet book. We compare celebrity diets in magazines. First, we were told that low-fat products were great, now they are not. It can be really confusing when trying to determine how you should eat for optimal health and weight. While some people do really well on certain diets, others may not. Because of bio-individuality, there is no one-size-fits-all nutritional lifestyle. Keto may not work for everyone, just like any other diet.

However, we can say factually that the low-fat diet myth has been debunked. Science has shown that it is not fat that is the enemy, it is sugar. Carbs, starches, processed sugar and other processed additives and synthesized foods are doing our bodies more harm than good.

While many people lose plenty of weight by drinking diet soda and overly-processed low-carb meal bars, their diet is not sustainable. This is why most diets fail and why we must differentiate between a diet and a nutritional lifestyle. Diets are a temporary fix. You cannot eat meal bars and diet soda for the rest of your life. The chemicals, additives and overall lack of nutrients will eventually make you incredibly sick. Not only that, but **your body will become nutritionally deficient**.

Food is like gasoline and your body is a vehicle. What happens when you use cheap gasoline to fill it? Yes, it will run for a while but it surely won't be long before you start experiencing problems. Before you know it, you're listening to the mechanic lecture you on using cheap gasoline.

The keto diet is the good gasoline. The stuff that has the engine cleaners and highest-quality petroleum. You don't want your car to run for a few hundred miles, you want it to run for hundreds of thousands. Think of your body in the same way. You want to be healthy, free of chronic illness and at a healthy weight and muscle mass, not just thinner.

There are other diets similar to keto but are not as popular. The reason for this is because they take more work, commitment and dedication. It takes much more care and thought to construct a great meal than to grab a low-fat sub from the sandwich shop or a low-fat can of soup off the shelf. But which will have the greater payoff? Fad diets and nutrient-deficient diet foods are a sure-fire way to fall off the wagon.

Your body can only go so long without nutrients before you wind up bingeing on sugar and fat in desperation. And once you have binged, you of course want to give up on the diet. On the contrary, the paleo diet, the Mediterranean diet, the Eastern diet are all fantastic, sustainable, whole-foods based lifestyles that will guarantee you a lifetime of health if you commit to it.

Do not let my words scare you off! **Going keto isn't *hard*, it is a *journey*.** Once you know what to eat, eating will be a breeze. The weight will melt off right before your eyes and you will feel the best you have ever felt – and very quickly! Along with a detailed shopping list and meal plan, I will include loads of keto-hacks and tips to make the transition as comfortable and simple as possible. You will be in ketosis before you can finish this book!

Chapter Two
Getting Started

Know your macros!

Macronutrients (or "macros") are three categories of nutrients that make up the caloric content of food. These three categories are fat, protein and carbohydrates. Every person has different macro measurements depending on their measurements and what their goals are. For example, a person who wants to build muscle is going to require more protein than a person who is trying to lose weight or maintain muscle mass. **Your macros will be the blueprint for your nutritional choices.**

The math and formulas are quite tricky. In a nutshell, you first determine what your daily caloric intake should be. From there, you figure out what percentage of those calories should be fat, protein and carbs. All of these numbers depend on not just your weight and height, but your age, activity level, BMI (Body Mass Index or body fat) and what your goals are.

The average macros for an average person would be 60-75% fat, 15-30% protein and 5-10% carbs. Carbs should never be more than 50g a day at most, but ideally, especially for weight loss, carbs would be under 30g a day. Of those carbs, 10-15g should be from vegetables, 5-10g should be from nuts and seeds and 5-10g should be from fruit.

There are 4 calories per gram of carbohydrates. Therefore, if our carb limit for the day is 20 net carbs, we multiply the two numbers and get 80 calories. So, 80 of our daily calories should come from carbs.

Protein

Many, if not most, diets push protein. For example, the Adkins diet calls for a high amount of protein. The thinking behind this theory is that the more protein we have, the less hungry we get. However, there is such a thing as too much protein. Consuming too much protein, especially animal protein, can actually produce glucose which is the very thing we are trying to avoid. This spikes our blood sugar and boots us right out of ketosis.

Finding the perfect balance is key in maintaining or building muscle mass. Those trying to lose weight or maintain lean body mass want to aim for .6-.9g of protein per pound of lean body mass. To build muscle mass, the target will be between .8-1.2g of protein per pound. Those trying to build muscle Your lean body mass is your ideal body mass. Here is an example:

If I weigh 160 lbs. and my BMI is 30% (I am 30% body fat), I multiply my current weight by the percent body fat to determine that I have 48 lbs. of body fat.

To find my lean body mass, I will subtract 48 lbs. from 160 lbs. which means my lean body mass (or, target weight) is 112 lbs.

Since I want to slowly build a small amount of muscle, my protein will be .8g/lb. So, I multiply 112 (my LBM) by .8 and find that I need 89.6g of protein each day.

When I multiply 89.6 by 4 (calories), I learn that of my daily calories, 358.4 of them should be from protein.

This is when we discover that we can load up on the good fat! Going off the math we just did, since I have a lot of body fat to lose, I will probably have a target caloric intake of about 1,200/day. If we subtract my calories from carbs and protein, I am left with 761g of fat for the day!

However, this does not mean loading up on bacon and ice cream. Remember, your fat should be coming from nuts, seeds, oils, fatty fish, avocado and MCT oil.

How do I figure out my macros? While you could do all the figuring, measuring and math by hand, if you can Google then you can figure it all out in a matter of seconds. There are plenty of great websites that allow you to plug in your numbers and get your results. You can simply look up "keto macro calculators" or you can check out my favorites:

Dream Shape: **www.mydreamshape.com/keto-calculator**

Kotoite Buddy:
www.ketodietapp.com/Blog/page/KetoDiet-Buddy

Food: The Good, The Bad and The Fatty

The easiest way to get going with a completely new way of eating is with a clear-cut list of do's and don'ts so I am happy to break these down for you. From here you can make grocery lists and plan meals accordingly.

The beauty of the keto diet is that because it is whole foods-based and low-glycemic, we won't be counting calories. Calories are energy and we will be getting our energy from fat, not from protein bars and rice, so we will be counting a lot of carbs, some protein, and a little bit of fat. However, because we're going to be chowing down on loads of good, healthy fats, it will be extremely difficult to go overboard with fat.

Here is a solid list of foods for you to get a good grasp on what to eat and what to avoid.

Fat/Oil:

Omega-3's and Omega-6's: Wild-caught salmon, tuna, trout, and other fatty fish.

Saturated/Monounsaturated fat: Nuts and seeds, especially almonds, pumpkin, etc. Nut butters are also an excellent source of both protein and fat and can be quite versatile. (But stay away from peanuts!), avocado, eggs, coconut oil, MCT oil, butter, olive oil, red palm oil, avocado oil, macadamia oil, ghee, cacao butter, etc.

Keep in mind, when cooking with fats/oils, if you are going to be frying or using them at high heat, make sure you are choosing the right oil. For example, vegetable oils like olive, flax, etc. will oxidize and lose their essential fatty acids. Fats like ghee and coconut oil do much better at high heat. Another use for nuts and seeds are flours! Subbing almond flour or ground flax seed for traditional flours and breading will cut the carbs and up the protein.

Protein: Fish and shellfish, eggs, meat, pork, poultry, bacon and sausage, nuts and nut butters. There are many vegetables that contain protein as well. Dark, leafy greens and avocado also have protein. Beans and legumes are super high in protein but can also be high in carbs so these should be used sparingly.

Veggies: Believe it or not, some veggies can be quite starchy and sugary. One trick is to stick to veggies that grow above ground. Avoid potatoes and other tubers. Some great keto-approved vegetables are: asparagus, avocado, olives, broccoli, carrots, cauliflower, celery, cucumbers, green beans, mushrooms, onions, bell peppers, pickles, dark, leafy greens, various squash and tomatoes. Fermented vegetables are a great addition to a keto diet! Pickles and sauerkraut are fabulous for your health and digestive system.

Dairy: Many keto-dieters opt for minimal dairy or skip it all together. Dairy products can very easily be full of sugar, carbs and additives and aren't great for digestion. Dairy can sometimes be blamed for acne, allergies and mucus issues, too. However, a reasonable amount of high quality, organic (and raw, if possible) dairy can be beneficial, especially in a keto lifestyle.

Some good dairy foods are: heavy whipping cream, both hard and soft cheese, sour cream, cottage cheese and full-fat Greek yogurt. Make sure all your dairy products are full-fat for two reasons. The first is that low-fat products are processed and usually loaded with fillers and sugar. The second reason is because you need the fat!

Fluids: Good news! Coffee is keto! So many diets encourage cutting the coffee, but it's A-Okay with a keto lifestyle. Of course, moderation is key with any source of caffeine and coffee can cause dehydration which you want to avoid while living keto. Staying hydrated is key as water flushes our system of toxins, helps with digestion and keeps us feeling fuller.

Drinking sparkling water with a squeeze of citrus is a delicious substitute for sodas and other sugary drinks and keeps you hydrated. Tea is wonderful, too. The rule of thumb is that you should drink half your body weight in ounces of water. I would recommend doing that, plus one more 8 oz. glass of water just to be sure. Your car won't run without oil, just like your body will shut down without water!

Vegan, vegetarian, pescetarian, ovo-lacto-tarian – what if I don't eat everything?!

You may, in your research, hear or read that avoiding meat and animal products while going keto is nearly impossible. Don't get discouraged because this is simply not true! There is a huge movement for going without animal products and it can be done quite easily. The trickiest part will be ensuring you get enough protein without going over your carb limit and this will just take some creativity on your part.

Non-GMO tofu, pumpkin seeds, almonds, and chia seeds are great examples of vegan low-carb, protein-dense options. Oils, olives, MCT oil, coconut milk and other nut butters are perfect for a vegan keto lifestyle.

How do I know if I'm in ketosis?

There are many natural indicators that your body is in ketosis. There are the obvious signs like keto flu, decreased appetite, increased focus and energy, suppressed appetite, etc.

But to know for sure, you can simply purchase urine strips at your local pharmacy. These will detect ketones in your urine. If you are shedding ketones, that means that you are producing more than enough and are in ketosis. Ketones can also be present in your breath which can be slightly stinky but treatable.

Chapter Three
Meal Plan

In order to make your transition into ketosis easier, I have included a two-week meal plan along with a grocery list. While there are thousands of terrific keto recipes out there, it is better to keep your meals simple with only a few ingredients in each meal. Often when attempting a new culinary lifestyle, people make the mistake of picking ingredients that they have never used and have no idea how to cook or use.

This is a sure-fire way to give up on your diet as soon as you start it. When cooking is frustrating and difficult, it makes us feel like we have failed. If we fail at cooking, we will definitely fail at eating and might as well give up. I want you to succeed and by sticking to this light and simple plan, you will absolutely succeed – and feel like a whole new person!

A Note on Organics

It is now common knowledge that organic is better. Free of chemicals and GMOs and much fresher than conventional produce, the organic choice is clearly the best. However, our budgets don't always allow for this. But don't fret! I am including a list of the must-haves for organic choices so that even if you can't go completely organic, you can make sure that you are still avoiding the worst offenders.

The "dirty dozen" are the twelve foods you should always buy organic. The following foods tested positive for anywhere between 47-67 chemicals:

- celery
- peaches
- strawberries
- apples
- domestic blueberries
- nectarines
- sweet bell peppers
- spinach, kale and collard greens
- cherries
- potatoes
- imported grapes
- lettuce

This brings us to the "clean fifteen" – the foods that you can buy that have little to no chemicals:

- onions
- avocado
- corn
- pineapples
- mango
- sweet peas
- asparagus

- kiwi
- cabbage
- eggplant
- cantaloupe
- watermelon
- grapefruit
- sweet potatoes
- sweet onions

However, when it comes to meat, dairy and eggs, grass-fed and organic should be the standard. Factory farmed meat is loaded with anti-biotics and the animals are often fed GMO corn and wheat products which, of course, transfers to the meat/milk/eggs which will end up in our bodies if consumed. Most conventional dairy products (cheese, milk, butter, etc.) also contain sugar, food dyes and other chemicals.

According to Dr. Toni Bark of The Center for Disease Prevention and Reversal, studies at Stanford University showed that *"antibiotic resistant microbes were more prevalent in meat from conventionally raised animals. This is huge (and obvious) as antibiotic resistance accounts for much morbidity and mortality in this country and is a growing concern".*

Do the best you can for your body, but do not stress or feel like a failure if you aren't in a position to go all-organic. As long as you are feeding your body the fuel it needs, you will certainly get better results than what you have now!

I have not included all of the kitchen "staples" in the recipes and lists. Many of the fats can be subbed per your own preferences. For example, you can alternate olive, avocado, coconut oils and butter. They are all under 1 carb and can be interchanged.

Here is a quick list of staples:

- Sour cream
- Dijon mustard
- Fat (olive oil, butter, ghee, coconut oil, etc.)
- Sea salt (Himalayan Pink Salt is preferred)
- Pepper
- Seasonings (paprika, garlic, etc.)
- Citrus juices or fresh citrus (lemon and lime)
- Mayonnaise
- MCT oil (can be taken as a supplement or added to food)
- Vegetable, chicken and other bone broths

Now let's get to the food!

Grocery List – Week One

- Eggs
- Cream Cheese
- Whole fat plain Greek yogurt
- Shredded mozzarella cheese
- Shredded cheddar or Mexican blend cheese
- 92% lean grass-fed ground beef
- Pork breakfast sausage (grass-fed)
- Lox
- Organic chicken breast
- Berries (blueberries, strawberries, etc.)
- Dried coconut (unsweetened) for snacking
- Cucumber
- Mixed greens (kale, spinach, chard, etc.)
- Spinach
- Lentils (White or red – whichever you prefer)
- Broccoli
- Cauliflower
- Macadamia nuts
- Almonds
- Cashews
- Flax seeds
- Green olives
- Diced tomatoes
- 1-2 lemons
- Canned pink salmon

- Spaghetti squash
- Tomato sauce (sugar-free)
- Avocadoes
- Nut butter (Cashew or almond)
- Extra virgin olive oil
- Avocado oil
- Salmon filet
- Bacon (grass-fed)
- Sliced deli ham
- Sliced provolone
- Roasted pumpkin seeds
- Asparagus
- Pork chop

Day One (31 carbs/55g protein):

Breakfast : Scramble two eggs in coconut oil with ¼ c. green olives and ¼ c. diced tomatoes

Lunch: Salad — Put together 3 c. leafy greens, 3 oz. sliced avocado, 3 oz. canned pink salmon, 1 oz. flax seeds and toss with 2 tbsp. olive oil and a squeeze of lemon juice.

Snack : 3.5 oz. plain Greek yogurt with ¼ c. berries

Dinner: Preheat your oven to 375. Take a spaghetti squash and slice it in half the long way. Scoop out the seeds and "guts" then drizzle with olive oil and sprinkle with salt and pepper. Place in a baking dish flat side down and bake for 35-45 minutes. In the meantime, brown 1 oz. 92% lean green beef in a pan then add ½ c. tomato sauce and seasonings (basil, oregano, garlic) and simmer until meat is cooked through. When the squash is finished, take it out and scrape the center with a fork into a bowl the long way. Strands of "spaghetti" will fall into the bowl. Continue scraping until all squash is in the bowl. Add your meat sauce and sprinkle with 1 oz. shredded mozzarella.

Day Two (31 carbs/55g protein):

Breakfast : 1.5 oz. pork breakfast sausage sautéed in the pan with 2 eggs (any way) and ½ c. berries.

Lunch : 10 oz. sliced cucumber topped with 4 oz. lox and 2 tbsp. cream cheese

Snack : 1 oz. dried coconut, unsweetened with 1 oz. macadamia nuts

Dinner : Add 1 c. veggie broth to saucepan and bring to a boil. Add ½ c. lentils and return to a boil then let it simmer with a lid on until all broth is absorbed (about 15 minutes). Sautee ½ c. broccoli and 1 c. cauliflower in pan with 1-2 tbsp. coconut oil and 1 garlic clove. Toss lentils and veggies together to enjoy.

Day Three (28 carbs/50g protein):

Breakfast : Fry 2 slices bacon and 2 eggs, scrambled then top eggs with 1 oz. shredded cheddar cheese

Lunch : Ham + provolone roll ups: Put 1 oz. deli sliced ham together with 1 oz. sliced provolone and roll plus ½ c. strawberries on the side.

Snack: 1 oz. cashews with 1 oz. dried coconut, unsweetened

Dinner: Sautee 4 oz. salmon fillet in 1-2 tbsp. coconut oil. When fish is finished (about 5-8 minutes), remove from pan and add 1 c. spinach. Cook spinach until wilted. Squeeze fresh lemon juice on fish and spinach.

Day Four (39 carbs/60g protein)

Breakfast : 3.5 oz. whole Greek yogurt topped with ½ c. berries, 1 oz. almonds and 1 tbsp. chia seeds

Lunch: Salad: Toss together 3 c. mixed greens with ¼ c. onion, 4 oz. bell pepper, 2 oz. carrots and 1 oz. sliced roasted chicken breast and drizzle with 2 tbsp. olive oil and squeeze of lemon.

Snack 1 oz. almonds, 1 oz. macadamia nuts and ½ oz. dried coconut, unsweetened

Dinner Preheat oven to 425. Take 4 oz. salmon fillet and drizzle with olive oil, pink salt and dill. Toss 1 c. asparagus in a bowl with olive oil and pink salt. Add salmon and asparagus to baking pan and bake for 8-10 minute (until fish is flaky). Sprinkle salmon and asparagus with 1 oz. parmesan cheese to enjoy.

Day Five (29 carbs/59g protein):

Breakfast: Add 2 tbsp. coconut oil to pan. Put 2 eggs, 6 oz. fresh spinach and ½ a tomato, diced, into pan. Scramble and cook until eggs are done. Add 3 oz. sliced avocado to enjoy

Lunch: Add 1 can tuna to a bed of 3 c. mixed greens with ½ c. white onion and ½ c. chopped celery and drizzle with 2-3 tbsp. olive oil and a squeeze lemon juice

Snack: ½ c. berries with 3.5 oz. whole Greek yogurt

Dinner: Sautee 1 medium pork chop seasoned with pink salt, pepper and pinch of paprika in a pan with 1 clove garlic and 2 tbsp. coconut oil. Steam 1 c. asparagus in saucepan by filling the bottom of the pan with water (about 1 inch.) and place steamer rack in the pan with asparagus on top and cover. Cook until asparagus is tender. Finish asparagus with a squeeze of lemon juice.

Day Six (41 carbs/83g protein):

Breakfast: In frying pan, cook 1.5 oz. pork sausage, 1 sliced tomato and 1 small sliced onion. Remove from pan when cooked and add 1 egg. Cook egg as desired.

Lunch: Ham roll-ups: 3 oz. sliced deli ham divided and stuffed with 10 oz. cucumber and 3 oz. avocado

Snack: ½ c. cottage cheese with sliced bell pepper

Dinner: Brown 4 oz. 92% ground beef in a pan then drain the fat. Add taco seasoning and cook until meat is done. Serve loose (no tortillas) and top with ½ c. onion, ½ c. bell pepper, 2 tbsp. sour cream and sprinkle of Mexican blend cheese.

Day Seven (29 carbs/67g protein)

Breakfast: Mix 2 eggs, ½ c. spinach, 2 diced tomatoes, already-cooked bacon in a bowl then split into two coffee mugs. Microwave 1-2 minutes and service with 3 oz. sliced avocado on top.

Lunch: Salad: Combine 1 c. mixed greens with 3 oz. avocado, 2 hard-boiled eggs, sliced, and ¼ c. onion. Drizzle with 2 tbsp. olive oil and lemon juice to taste.

Snack: ½ C. berries with 1 oz. cashews

Dinner: In food processor, combine ½ c. walnuts, 2 tbsp. maple syrup and ½ tbsp. Dijon mustard until finely chopped. Slather mixture onto 3 oz. salmon fillet and sauté in a pan with olive oil. Cook about 5-8 minutes, until fish can be flaked with a fork.

Now we can start week two, before that remember that if you are enjoying this book, you can leave a quick review on Amazon.

It would be much appreciated!

And now to our meal plan for the second week!

Grocery List – Week Two

This week we will have a little more fun with some of the recipes. Week one was very simple and basic so that it can be achievable to even the most novice of cooks. While week two will still be quite simple, the recipes will call for a bit more creativity so that we can avoid boredom.

Now that you have a solid understanding of how and what to cook, feel free to start experimenting a bit! Try a variety of flavors and seasoning as this will be the easiest way to transform your meals. Note that many of this week's meals call for items that we used last week so if you still have something leftover, you don't need to buy it again so you can adjust this grocery list accordingly.

Grocery List

- 2-3 salmon fillets
- Walnuts, cashews, almonds
- Eggs
- Mixed salad greens
- Fresh spinach
- Shrimp
- Avocados
- Onions
- Tomatoes
- Zucchini
- Spaghetti squash
- Bell peppers
- Boneless, skinless chicken breast
- Fresh kale
- Green olives
- Feta cheese
- Sliced Swiss and mozzarella cheese
- Sliced deli ham
- Pickles
- Fresh berries
- Plain, whole fat Greek yogurt
- Heavy cream
- Bacon
- Pork sausage
- Polish sausage

- 1 ribeye steak
- Brussels sprouts
- Broccoli
- String cheese
- Ground beef
- Shredded Mexican cheese
- Cream cheese
- Head of green cabbage
- Cottage cheese
- Deviled eggs (store-bought or home-made)
- Heavy cream
- Mushrooms
- Cucumber
- Hummus

Day One (25 carbs/76g protein)

Breakfast: Whisk 2 eggs and add to hot skillet with 1 tbsp. coconut oil. Allow eggs to cook for 1 minutes then add ½ c. broccoli. Once eggs are cooked through, add 1 slice Swiss cheese on top of broccoli then fold eggs into an omelet.

Lunch: Salad: Combine 2 c. leafy greens, 2 oz. cooked shrimp, 3 oz. avocado, ¼ c. chopped onion, ½ c. diced tomato drizzled with olive oil, lime juice and cilantro.

Snack: ½ c. mixed berries with 1 oz. roasted pecans.

Dinner: 1 6 oz. boneless, skinless chicken breast sautéed in olive oil and topped with 2 slices tomato, 2-4 basil leaves, 1 slice mozzarella. Drizzle with balsamic dressing.

Day Two (18 carbs/45g protein)

Breakfast: Take 1 avocado, halved, and scoop out center to make a good-sized divot. Crack 1 egg into each hole and place avocados in baking pan. Bake 15 minutes at 425 degrees then sprinkle with choice of seasoning.

Lunch: 1 can of tuna mixed with 1 tbsp. mayonnaise, ½ tsp. Dijon mustard, ¼ c. celery and 2 tbsp. chopped onions. Slice the top off one large or two small tomatoes and scoop out the seeds and insides then stuff with the tuna mixture.

Snack: 1 cup green olives with 1 oz. feta cheese

Dinner: Grill 1-4 oz. rib eye steak. While steak is grilling, sauté ½ c. sliced mushrooms in 2 tbsp. butter and 2 tbsp. heavy cream. Cook until desired thickness. Then steam 1. C chopped broccoli in a sauce pan. When steak is done, top with mushroom mixture and enjoy with broccoli.

Day Three (17 carbs/88g protein)

Breakfast: Mix 2 eggs, 2 tbsp. heavy cream and 1 oz. chopped onion and scramble in skillet with 1-2 tbsp. coconut oil. Enjoy with 4 slices of bacon, fried in skillet.

Lunch: Add 3 oz. grilled chicken breast strips over 3 cups mixed greens, 1 celery stick, chopped, and drizzle with olive oil and lemon juice.

Snack: 2 mozzarella string cheese sticks with 1 oz. almonds

Dinner: Toss 1 c. Brussels sprouts in olive oil and sea salt, roast in oven at 425 for 20-30 minutes. Sautee 3 oz. salmon fillet drizzled with olive oil and pinch of garlic powder. Serve a side salad of 1 c. mixed greens and 3 oz. avocado drizzled with olive oil and lemon or lime juice.

Day Four (33 carbs/63g protein)

Breakfast: 3.5 oz. Greek yogurt with 1 oz. chia seeds and ½ c. blueberries

Lunch: 2 oz. deli ham, separated and filled with 2 tbsp. cream cheese and pickle spears

Snack: 2 oz. Kale chips with olive oil and lemon juice. These can usually be bought at any grocery store, but can also be made by tossing kale leaves in olive oil, sea salt and lemon juice and baking in oven at 100 for 1-2 hours, depending on their moisture.

Dinner: 3 oz. chicken breast strips sautéed with 1 c. bell pepper strips, ½ c. onions in olive oil and fajita seasoning topped with 1 oz. Mexican cheese

Day Five (26 carbs/71g protein)

Breakfast: 2 eggs scrambled with 1 oz. feta and ½ a zucchini, chopped, and topped with 3 oz. sliced avocado.

Lunch: Bun less burger: 4 oz. ground beef grilled or sautéed and topped with 1 oz. Swiss cheese, onion slices, 1 bacon strip, halved, mustard and mayo.

Snack: ½ c. blueberries with 1 oz. almonds

Dinner: Sautee 2 oz. shrimp and 1 oz. sliced pork sausage in coconut oil and 1-2 cloves of garlic. Add ½ c. shredded cabbage to the skillet and cook for another 1-2 minutes then enjoy.

Day Six (31 carbs/72g protein)

Breakfast: 2 pork sausage links, sliced, with 1 c. mixed onion, zucchini, red pepper and squash sautéed all together in 1-2 tbsp. butter.

Lunch: 4 deviled eggs (store bought). These can be made at home as well by hard-boiling 2 eggs. Peel and slice each egg in half then scoop out the yolks into a mixing bowl. Add a squirt of mayo and a squirt of mustard and combine. Return yolk mixture to egg whites and top with paprika.

Snack: ½ c. cottage cheese with ½ c. olives

Dinner: Sautee sliced polish sausage in 1-2 tbsp. olive oil, garlic and ¼ c. chopped onion. Add 1 c. shredded cabbage with 2 tbsp. red wine vinegar and cook for a few more minutes (until cabbage is slightly tender). Add salt, pepper and paprika to taste.

Day Seven (29 carbs/70g protein)

Breakfast: Combine 2 eggs with 1 tbsp. pesto and 1 tbsp. sour cream then scramble in skillet with 1-2 tbsp. coconut oil. Enjoy with 2 slices of fried bacon.

Lunch: 1 avocado, halved, and stuff with 1 can of tuna with 1 tbsp. mayonnaise.

Snack: 10 oz. sliced cucumber topped with 1 oz. hummus (for dipping).

Dinner: 3 oz. shrimp sautéed in 1 tbsp. butter, 2 tbsp. olive oil and 2 cloves of garlic. Serve over 1 c. spaghetti squash (recipe in previous week) with 1 c. steamed spinach

Fat Bombs

Whenever I mention fat bombs, people tend to giggle and are quite intrigued to learn more. Fat bombs are a keto dieter's best friend. Since the goal is to get our bodies to burn fat instead of carbs, we need to replace those carby snacks with fatty snacks and these little treats are the easiest way to make sure we are doing just that. These are perfect for breakfast, an afternoon snack and before or after a workout. They are loaded with good fat and basically zero carbs so they won't screw up your macros.

Fat bombs usually consist of only 2-4 ingredients and can be made in ice trays or mini muffin pans so you can keep them fresh and pop one or two when you are in need of energy. While fat bombs are usually sweet, you can make savory ones, too. You can use a base of either coconut oil, coconut butter or other nut butters. Avoid peanut butter as it is high in carbs and sugar and stick to almond and other low-carb nuts. Fat bombs should be kept in an air-tight container in the fridge or freezer and can last for 1-2 weeks this way.

There are three essential parts that make up a fat bomb.

1. Fat
2. Flavor
3. Texture/Add-ins

Using this template, you can start mixing and matching ingredients to find your favorites! Just mix, freeze and eat!

Here are a few of my favorite fat bomb recipes:

- Coconut oil (liquefied), unsweetened cranberry juice and cacao
- Coconut oil, lemon juice and vanilla
- Olive oil, honey, cinnamon and vanilla
- Almond butter, coconut oil, chai spice and vanilla

Other delicious mix-ins:

- Crushed pistachios
- Shredded coconut
- Cacao nibs
- Green tea matcha
- Berries
- Coconut milk
- Cashew cream
- Sea salt
- Tahini (for a savory kick!)

Dessert

You may have noticed that I did not include sweets or dessert in the two-week meal plan. And yes, I did this purposefully. Usually when we are beginning a new nutritional lifestyle, we have some bad eating habits and food addictions to get under control.

Sugar is an addictive substance and I believe that it is better to quit it cold turkey rather than tapering off. It makes the process of detoxing a lot faster, meaning you will start feeling better (and losing weight) a whole lot sooner.

However, if you need your after-dinner treat, I strongly advise you to stick with fat bombs, raw cacao or dark chocolate or a spoonful of nut butter. I have often found that a warm cup of herbal tea after dinner kicks those sweet cravings right through the door, but everyone has to find what works for them. I will admit that I have resorted to what I like to call my **"emergency fat bomb."** This is a fat bomb that takes no prep time so in the event of a sweet attack, you can have it in your mouth faster than it would take to scoop the ice cream!

Emergency Fat Bomb:

Tablespoon of almond or cashew butter with a tiny drizzle of honey and sprinkle of cinnamon or cacao powder.

Because of the thick nut butter, it will actually take you awhile to get this little treat down and make it much more satisfying than it sounds.

Chapter Four
Keto Kitchen Hacks

You've just read through your two-week meal plan and your probably feeling overwhelmed and rightly so. That is a lot of food, a lot of cooking and a lot of money in two weeks! How can you possibly do that? Here's how:

Make it your own.

I intentionally created a new recipe for every single meal so that you will have 42 different meals plus 14 snacks to choose from. Everyone has different budgets, tastes, preferences and schedules so do what works for you. Eliminate the meals that don't sound good to you and replace them with your own creation or, even better, with leftovers!

Let's just get straight to the kitchen hacks so you can adjust to your new lifestyle!

Track your macros

Now that your kitchen is stocked with a bounty of keto-safe foods, you are free to play around with the recipes and ingredients. Just make sure you stick to your macros! You can find a plethora of macro charts online that breakdown carbs, fat and protein for just about every ingredient there is.

My favorite go-to for nutritional data is "SELFNutrition Data" (http://nutritiondata.self.com). This website is loaded with charts, calculators and nutritional data that will keep you on track. You can plug in your ingredients and find the macros for an array of serving sizes.

The site also generates lists of food recommendations per the dietary needs you input. For example, if you type in "Low-carbohydrates" it will pull up a list of low-carb options and their nutritional data. You can add in other specifics as well and create an entire, personalized keto list for yourself complete with data.

You will find yourself referencing these charts a lot in the beginning but as you get the hang of it, you will have it all in your head and know exactly where you stand for the day!

It is a good idea to keep a small notebook or journal with you for the first few weeks or months so that you don't go over or under your daily macros. You might think you can track everything in your head, but by snack time you've lost count. Do yourself a favor and make it simple for your brain.

Another great way to track your macros in the kitchen is by labelling! Take one day a week to prep your meals and snacks and divide them up into individual servings in baggies or Tupperware. You can then label each one with a marker to display each container's macros! You can also label containers of nuts, seeds, yogurt and other portioned foods.

Meal Prep

I'm sure you have heard of meal prepping by now. It's become a popular way to make your meals ahead for the week. Plan your menu, grocery shop, then cook and divvy it all up. This will help you avoid eating out at lunch time and will save you loads of time and energy. You can just pop the Tupperware into the microwave and you're done! Take them to work with you and you won't have to cook in the evening which means you won't have an excuse to order that pizza or grab a burger.

Bulk Cooking

Cooking in bulk goes hand in hand with meal prep. I like to make a huge pot of soup or cauliflower rice that will last me a few days. This way I am not reaching for a bag of chips or bowl of cereal and instead am warming up something good. By pre-cooking large quantities of vegetables or meat, you are saving yourself a great amount of time. Make a big pot of cauliflower rice cooked in vegetable broth and you can use it for many different meals throughout the week! You can add some to a veggie stir fry one day and to a curry the next. Anything you can cook ahead in bulk, do it.

Seasoning and Salt

Seasoning and flavor can make or break a healthy diet. Many people begin eating healthy with boring meals like dry chicken and bland steamed broccoli. No wonder they wind up bingeing on chips! Your pantry staples should include a large variety of seasonings and spices, including salt! While many people believe that salt should be used sparingly, this just isn't true. Table salt has basically no nutritional value and is not good for you. However, true salts are a wonderful supplement.

Salt is even more important in a ketogenic diet! **Himalayan Pink Salt** is probably the best salt you can buy. It is just as cheap as any other salt, but comes with huge nutritional value. Pink salt has no additives or iodine (like table salt) and contains lots of important minerals and magnesium (which most people are deficient in!). It helps balance the pH of your cells and can keep your blood sugar low. I know some keto people who actually carry pink salt in their purse for restaurant meals!

The beauty of seasoning is that it can transform any meal. You can take some plain old chicken and veggies and make it whatever you want. From Mexican style to curries to Asian, a little seasoning will go a long way. Also, cooking with broth adds loads of flavor to any dish. Making your own broth is quite easy and the healthiest way to go. Unless you are an experienced chef, keeping your meals simple is going to be key to your success and seasonings will keep those simple meals tasting extravagant and exciting.

Some must-haves in the pantry are:

- Himalayan Pink Salt
- Pepper
- Yellow curry
- Oregano
- Basil (fresh is best!)
- Paprika
- Hot sauce
- Bragg's liquid aminos
- Turmeric
- Chili powder
- Cumin
- Dill
- Lemon and lime juice
- Tahini

Keto Coffee

You may have heard about a new fad where people put butter in their coffee and if you have I am sure you wondered why the heck anyone would do that? The answer is pretty simple: because it is quite possibly the perfect keto combo. Most people love coffee and have a cup or two in the morning and afternoon for a boost of energy.

Coffee increases focus and is full of anti-oxidants and fat-burning polyphenols, too! The anti-oxidants in it fight liver disease and cancer, Parkinson's and type 2 diabetes. As long as you're not going overboard, coffee can be incredibly beneficial.

So imagine how powerful that little cup of joe would be if we added our new best friend, fat, to it! Many people opt for grass-fed, organic butter but choosing MCT oil is going to be the most beneficial.

When we add a tablespoon or two of fat to our coffee, we immediately get a boost of sustained energy. It also jump starts our metabolism for the day and increases fat-burning throughout the day. For those who practice *intermittent fasting* (which we will get to very soon), keto coffee is the perfect way to get through the day until meal time.

First, let's talk about MCT oil and supplements before we go any further!

MCT Oil and Supplements

MCT's (Medium Chain Triglycerides) are pretty much the superhero of fats. They are a fatty acid that is found in coconut oil and improve brain function, metabolism and boost ketone production. MCTs also improves metabolism and helps to maintain healthy blood sugar levels. Because MCTs don't require bile to be broken down, they are immediately converted into ketones (energy). Basically, they act like carbs in that they provide immediate energy but they don't raise blood sugars or insulin nor do they become stored fat. When you consume MCTs, you are giving your body and brain straight ketones.

They also aid in the absorption of nutrients like calcium and magnesium and work as a natural appetite suppressant! The list of benefits keeps growing.

MCTs can be found primarily in coconut oil, palm oil, and raw, organic dairy products like ghee, raw milk and kefir. If you are trying to avoid dairy you can stick to coconut oil but if you can't tolerate dairy, you can also do grass-fed ghee as it is highly-tolerated.

Or, you can go the easiest route which is to purchase a high-quality MCT oil. Keep a bottle on your kitchen counter and a small bottle in your purse, car or gym bag to make sure you don't forget to take it. You can use this directly in coffee, food, green smoothies, with some broth or straight up. However you choose to get your MCTs, make sure you load up as this is a key component to a successful ketogenic diet.

Other Key Supplements

- Coconut oil- for good fat and MCTs.
- Omega-3 fish oil – in small amounts, fish oil can lower triglycerides and contains DHA, ALA and EPA, fatty acids necessary for brain function and overall health. It can also aid in weight loss.
- Caffeine – for energy and focus.
- Magnesium – many magnesium-rich foods are also higher in carbs so we tend to eat less when we go keto. Avocados,

yogurt and nuts are high in magnesium, but we may need to supplement also.
- Sodium + Potassium- When we lower our insulin, we also lower our sodium and potassium. Adding pink salt and consuming other naturally-salty foods helps maintain sodium levels.
- Greens/Superfoods – Spirulina lowers triglycerides and LDL (bad) cholesterol. The benefits of dark, leafy greens and superfoods are endless so adding a scoop of a high-quality greens supplement to our regimen can do wonders.
- Vitamin D – Vitamin D can only be gotten from sunshine absorption and some fatty fish and it is necessary for a multitude of our body's functions. Most people are deficient in D3 and should be supplementing. Have your levels checked before choosing a supplement.

Many of these supplements will also aid you if you succumb to the "keto flu" which we previously discussed in chapter one. Sodium, potassium and magnesium will all help to combat symptoms of the keto flu as it is usually a result of the drastic decline of these nutrients in our bodies. **Supplementing with veggie or bone broth the first few days will up your sodium and other nutrients and easy symptoms as well.**

Golden Milk

Another fabulous addition to your keto kitchen are the ingredients for Golden Milk. While you can find many recipes online, the easiest way is to either buy golden milk powder pre-mixed from your local health food store or making it yourself. Golden milk is a combination of turmeric, ginger, cinnamon, cardamom, black pepper, MCT or coconut oil in warm milk. (Raw dairy or nut milk will do just fine – just check the carb count on the nut milk!)

Golden milk aids in digestion, weight loss, reduces inflammation, boost the immune system and adds a bump of fat. This can also be a wonderful aid for the "keto flu" as it calms the stomach and is easy to digest. It gives a small boost of magnesium and potassium, too.

Here is a basic recipe:

2 c. milk of choice (coconut milk would be ideal)

1 tsp. turmeric

½ tsp. cinnamon

¼ tsp. ginger powder

¼ tsp. cardamom

Pinch of black pepper

Add coconut oil or MCT oil to taste

Heat all together and whisk, then enjoy!

It is very important to avoid any little mistake that could limit your progress, that is why I added this Kitchen Hacks section.

However if you want to know more about common mistakes many people make when following the diet you can check Chapter 4 of this detailed Guide I made on Keto:

Keto Guide:The Clear Guide to your Keto Path

Chapter Five
Tips for Maximizing and Maintaining a Keto Lifestyle

You now have a kitchen stocked with keto-approved foods, you have your meal plan, you have chosen some beneficial supplements and are ready to change your life! But before you dive in, I want to go into some in-depth discussions on how to maximize your new lifestyle. How many times have you tried and given up on a diet? If you haven't, then I'm sure you know at least one person who has done this.

Many times, people will start out with the right intentions, eager to lose weight and improve health. They might last a few days or even a few weeks before they "relapse" and give up. They might cave and eat a "bad" meal, which in turn makes them feel guilty, and these feelings of low self-esteem lead to more "bad" eating until they give up completely. There are many reasons for failing at a healthier lifestyle and in this chapter, we will walk through them to make sure that you will succeed.

We will also talk a bit about various issues that might arise, and touch on topics like how to get children involved in a keto lifestyle, holistic approaches to eating and fitness.

"Keto Flu"

Also known as the "induction flu", this is a very common occurrence when diving into a low-carb lifestyle. While not everyone is affected by keto flu, it is good to know about before beginning so that you can be prepared to combat the symptoms.

It is not actually the flu but it can definitely feel like it. Symptoms include: headaches, nausea, vomiting, brain fog, fatigue and sleepiness and can last anywhere from a day to a week and even two weeks in the most dramatic and rare cases. This is because our bodies are so used to carbs that we have become dependent on them almost like sugar, caffeine or any other physically-addictive substance.

You can look at the keto flu as a detox as our bodies are suddenly deprived of something that they have been running on for probably our entire lives. Our bodies are full of enzymes ready to burn glucose, but now we will be generating new enzymes that burn fat. This transition period is the keto flu.

Please do not let this deter you from going keto! I promise you, it is worth it. Plus, there is plenty you can do to ease your symptoms. Let's go through them so you can be ready:

- **Hydrate!** You are more than likely dehydrated as most people are. As I've mentioned before, you should aim to drink half your body weigh in ounces of water and then add a glass or two. Water is key to proper function, especially of

- **Get enough electrolytes.** Again, as I have mentioned in the previous chapter, when our insulin drops, so do our sodium, magnesium and potassium levels. These are electrolytes. But instead of reaching for a bottle of sugary, carby sports drinks, opt instead for **chicken, beef or veggie broth** or even add **bouillon** cubes to your water. There are, of course, plenty of over-the-counter supplements that provide electrolytes and magnesium as well.
- **Eat fat.** You can speed up the process of adjusting to burning fat instead of glucose by adding lots of fat. Add MCT oil to your broth and coffee or eat a spoonful of coconut or other nut butter. Many people actually do a broth and fat fast during the first few days of keto and this is something we will talk about next.
- **Ease up on protein.** Too much protein can create glucose which can slow down the process of transitioning to low-carb. This doesn't mean skip protein altogether, but keep it to a low-to-moderate amount the first day or two. Again, fasting can aid in this transition.

Remember that the keto flu won't last forever. The best way to get through it is to view it as a good thing! Your body is preparing itself to become a fat-burning machine and this is the first step. Once you have made it through, you will feel amazing. Most people report feeling clear-headed, energized, light and overall better than before they even began. There is a light at the end of the tunnel.

Intermittent Fasting

Fasting is a wonderful tool for the ketogenic lifestyle. There has long been belief that breakfast is the most important meal of the day because it boosts metabolism, improves focus and gives the body sustained energy. But what about those of us who aren't hungry in the morning or feel nauseous after eating first thing? Are our bodies wrong? The answer is no, it is perfectly normal.

There are benefits to intermittent fasting including: mental clarity, increased fat-burning (ketogenic state), better control over macros, and can help reduce over-eating.

Some people choose to begin their keto lifestyle with a 12-24 hour fast to get into a state of ketosis faster. This means limiting your intake to broth, water and fatty oils (MCT, coconut, etc.) to induce ketosis and speed up the transition.

Once in ketosis, it can be beneficial to create "eating windows." In other words, you might go 12-18 hours without eating and limit eating to the other 6-12 hours. During the "fasting" portion of the day (usually from sleep until afternoon or evening), you would stick to keto coffee, water, and/or broth. During the fasting portion, your body will burn stored fat so make sure you are replenishing with good fats throughout the day.

This could explain why some of us are not hungry in the morning! Our bodies could be naturally keto-adaptive, meaning our bodies feel better with intermittent fasting. The key is to do what is right for your lifestyle and your body.

Many athletes find fasted workouts to be more effective as well. As long as you are safe and hydrated, see what works for you. There is no one-size-fits-all diet.

Eating Out

Of course you are going to eat what is available to you which is why you want to make sure your kitchen is stocked with good options, meal prep and plan ahead. It is a good idea not only to meal prep but to keep snacks in your bag or car. Keeping a bag of nuts can save you from a slip-up. There are also plenty of keto-friendly options pretty much everywhere.

Many gas stations and pharmacies carry string cheese, deli meat snacks and even hard-boiled eggs or hummus in their refrigerated sections. But what do you do when invited out to a restaurant? We can't decline social events because of our nutritional lifestyle. Don't panic – there are plenty simple ways to make sure you stay on track even at the most indulgent of restaurants.

At almost all restaurants, the menu is customizable. What you see on the menu does not mean that is what you are limited to. At Mexican restaurants, ordering fajitas with no tortillas is an easy fix. Chinese menus often include meat or tofu and veggies, just ask them to hold the rice. Italian restaurants might seem impossible, but more often than naught there are options for items that include meat or eggplant and ask for vegetables instead of pasta. There are salad and soup options at almost every restaurant as well.

Of course, temptation might be an issue, especially in the first few weeks of eating keto. **A trick that I still use is to eat before you go.** Yes, it sounds funny but this trick has worked better for me than anything else. I often found myself too tempted while out and would tell myself "it will be okay this one time" but that is a slippery slope and often how most people wind up giving up on a healthy lifestyle.

You don't need to eat a full meal before going out to a restaurant, but eating just enough at home to take the edge off will do wonders. This way, when you are starting at a menu full of pasta, rice and bread, you are already pretty full so soup or salad will sound like just enough. This also will help prevent over-eating as happens so often, especially with such large portions usually being served.

Mindfulness

Mindfulness is an incredible tool for cultivating a healthy lifestyle. When we are aware not only of what we are eating, but how we are feeling and what our body needs, we can have more control and satisfaction with our good habits. For example, adjusting to less food can be psychologically difficult for many people.

Although our body says we are full, our brain still wants to eat more. This can be combative by eating mindfully. **Chew slowly, put your fork down between each bite, close your eyes and focus on the tastes as you eat each bite, think about how you are nourishing your body and what**

each food is doing for your body. Eating should be an enjoyable experience. We should not feel guilty or negative. By practicing mindful eating, we can combat those bad feelings.

Mindfulness can be applied to grocery shopping and cooking as well. When grocery shopping, take your time and touch and smell all the produce. Sample things. Look at things and think about all the wonderful things that food is going to do for you.

Make cooking and meal prepping an event or ritual. You are creating meals that are going to nourish your body and mind and transform your health. Again, take your time, focusing on how delicious each meal will be and praise yourself for making such good decisions for yourself. Think about how that meal is going to make you feel mentally and physically and get excited.

When we "go on a diet" without practicing mindfulness, we often get no enjoyment out of the restrictive eating process. Do not look at keto as restrictive. Instead, you are not allowing unhealthy, negative foods to harm your body any longer. You are fueling your body in a positive way and that is something to celebrate with every meal.

The Keto Family

If you have children and/or a partner, you might want to share your new nutritional lifestyle with them in hopes for a healthier, happier family. While there are contradictory opinions on whether or not keto is safe for kids, the bottom line is you have to decide what is right for you and your family.

Although children of a healthy weight digest sugar and carbs differently than us (they tend to burn them off rapidly as kids are constantly active), they can still benefit from a low-carb lifestyle just as adults do for all the same reasons. Healthy weight, sustained energy, low blood sugar, low cholesterol, reduced risk of cancer and type 2 diabetes and some studies have shown that a low-carb diet is effective in reversing epilepsy in children.

Many parents struggle with getting their children to adapt to healthy eating habits and allow their children to hate vegetables and other healthy options. Remember that, as their parent, *you* ultimately decide what goes in their bodies and what does not. If you and your child's doctor feel that a keto diet would be safe, there are plenty of resources online with kid-friendly keto recipes. Getting your kids excited and involved will be the best way to transition them to a keto lifestyle with you.

Let them pick out items at the grocery store and explain to them *why* that item is good (or bad) and what it will do for their bodies. Let them partake in the cooking/meal prepping process. Encourage them to make good choices for themselves and positively reinforce when they do. It may take time, but with encouragement, involvement and consistency, your kids will learn to live keto with you.

Your children will learn everything from you, including eating habits, so you must decide what kind of example you will set.

You are also more likely to succeed if your household is on the same page. The beauty of the keto diet is that it works for men and women. Men don't need to skimp on meat and cheese and a growing number of athletes and bodybuilders, male and female, are going keto.

Rally your partner or family for support and involvement – this will make your transition fun and exciting, and you will have a built-in support group right at home!

If you don't have people at home, ask a friend to jump in with you so you have an accountability partner. It does wonders to have someone to share successes and opportunities with especially if we struggle or "slip up", we can have a partner to help us get right back on the horse.

Other Support

There is an incredible amount of support all over the web. With low-carb growing in popularity, there are blogs, support groups, social media groups and online resources to keep you going. You can find tools, calculators, meal ideas and anything else you might need through a quick search online or in social media. Although you can go keto alone, it makes it a lot easier and more fun when you find encouragement and help along the way.

Conclusion

Hopefully by now you feel excited and prepared to begin your ketogenic journey. If you found the idea of keto or low-carb daunting, I hope you now see that it can be quite simple and achievable. Although it can be difficult to get started, if you follow these tips and guidelines and find the right support, you will succeed.

It is important to keep learning about the subject, the more you know about it the better you will apply the principles.

It could be beneficial for you to check a <u>detailed analysis of this diet here</u>: <u>Keto Guide:The Clear Guide to your Keto Path</u>.

The key takeaways are to have fun and be creative, make going keto fun and rewarding and develop a positive relationship between your body and mind.

I am glad you choose **The Keto Diet Made Simple** as your first step or as a guide to your new nutritional lifestyle, it might take time but I am confident that with this guide you will achieve your goals

Finally, <u>if you found this book useful,</u> I would really appreciate if you could <u>leave a quick review on Amazon,</u> Thank you!

Steven G. Canty

As I mentioned, the book <u>Keto Guide:The Clear Guide to your Keto Path</u> is a detailed guide that complement the book you have just read, focusing on certain aspects of the diet that I consider fundamental. Even the meal plan that it contains is just one week long but more in detail, as I show you in this extract and I leave you as **1 bonus** Meal Plan Day!

Preview Of "<u>Keto Guide: The Clear Guide to your Keto Path</u>"

Meal Plan Day 4

Breakfast: Smoked Salmon Sammie on Pumpkin Bread

This recipe needs 5 minutes to prepare, 10 minutes to cook and will make 2 servings.

- Fat: 82 percent
- Protein: 15 percent
- Carbs: 2 percent

What to Use-Bread

- Coconut oil (1 T)
- Pumpkin puree (1 can)
- Coconut oil (.25 cups)
- Apple sauce (.5 cups unsweetened)
- Eggs (3 large)
- Pumpkin seeds (.3 cups)
- Walnuts (.3 cups chopped)
- Coconut flour (1.25 cups)
- Almond flour (1.25 cups)
- Flax seeds (.5 cups)
- Psyllium husk (2 T powdered)
- Salt (1 tsp.)
- Baking powder (1 T)
- Pumpkin pie spice (2 T)

What to Use-Filling

- Chives (1 T chopped)
- Salmon (3 oz. smoked)
- Lettuce (1 oz.)
- Butter (2 T grass fed)
- Chili flakes (1 pinch)
- Butter (2 T grass fed)
- Pepper (to taste)
- Salt (to taste)
- Heavy whipping cream (2 T)
- Eggs (4 large)
- Egg (2 scrambled)

What to Do-Bread

- Start by making sure your oven is heated to 400 degrees F.
- Grease a bread pan (8 inches) using grass fed butter
- In a mixing bowl combine the walnuts, coconut flour, almond flour, flax seeds, psyllium powder, salt, baking powder and pumpkin pie spice and mix well.
- Mix in the pumpkin puree, coconut oil, apple sauce and eggs and combine thoroughly.
- Add the batter to the prepared baking dish and top with 1 T pumpkin seeds.
- Place the pan on the bottom rack in the oven and let it bake for 60 minutes. You will know it is finished when you can stick a knife in and it comes out clean.

What to Do-Sammie

- In a small bowl, combine the heavy whipping cream with the eggs and whisk well before seasoning as needed with pepper and salt.
- Add the butter to a frying pan before placing in the stove on top of a burner set to a medium heat. Once the butter has melted, add in the egg mixture and stir well prior to removing the frying pan from the stove. Add in the chili powder and mix well
- Add the results to two pieces of toasted pumpkin bread, top with lettuce, smoked salmon, chives and scrambled eggs.

Lunch: Keto Tuna Melt

This recipe needs 5 minutes to prepare, 15 minutes to cook and will make 1 serving.

- Fat: 75 percent
- Protein: 23 percent
- Carbs: 1 percent

What to Use- Bread

- Baking powder (.5 tsp.)
- Psyllium husk (.5 T powder)
- Salt (1 pinch)
- Cream cheese (4 oz.)
- Eggs (3)

What to Use-Filling

- Cheese (shredded 4 oz.)
- Garlic (.5 cloves minced)
- Lemon juice (.5 tsp.)
- Olive oil (1 can)
- Dill pickles (.25 cups chopped)
- Celery (1 stalk)
- Sour cream (.3 cups)

What to Do-Bread

- Start by making sure your oven is heated to 300 degrees F.
- Separate the eggs from their yolks and save both in separate bowls.
- Add salt to the whites and whisk well.
- Add the cream cheese to the yolks and mix well before adding in the baking powder and psyllium.
- Combine the two bowls and mix well before adding the results to a baking sheet so that it will form eight slices.
- Bake in the center of the oven for 25 minutes

What to Do-Filling

- Start by making sure your oven is heated to 350 degrees F.
- Combine all of the filling ingredients, minus the cheese, together in a bowl and mix well.
- Place two slices of bread onto a lined baking sheet and top with filling and finish with cheese.
- Bake 15 minutes.

Dinner: Italian Sausage with Vegetables

This recipe needs 10 minutes to prepare, 40 minutes to cook and will make 4 servings.

- Fat: 82 percent
- Protein: 13 percent
- Carbs: 4 percent

What to Use

- Olive oil (.25 cups)
- Italian sausage (1 lb.)
- Thyme (1 T dried)
- Black pepper (.25 T ground)
- Sea salt (.5 tsp.)
- Mozzarella cheese (.5 lbs. diced)
- Cherry tomatoes (.3 lbs. diced)
- Garlic (4 cloves chopped)
- Onion (2 chopped)
- Zucchini (1 small, sliced)
- Butter (1 oz. grass fed)

What to Do

- Start by making sure your oven is heated to 400 degrees F.
- Grease a baking dish.
- Add all of the vegetables to a baking dish before adding in the cheese amongst the results and top with the olive oil. Add in the sausage and season as needed.
- Place the baking dish into the oven and let it cook for 40 minutes.

You can find the rest of the book here!
Keto Guide: The Clear Guide to your Keto Path

Printed in Poland
by Amazon Fulfillment
Poland Sp. z o.o., Wrocław